Diabetes Mellitus (Ziabetus Shakri)
AN OVERVIEW

Adnan Mastan

BUMS, MD (Medicine),

FIII, DHI, DHM, DLU

Diabetes Mellitus (Ziabetus Shakri)
AN OVERVIEW

Name of the Book: Diabetes Mellitus (Ziabetus Shakri): An Overview

Name of the Author: Dr.Adnan Mastan

Published: August 2015

Edition: First

Note: As new information becomes available, changes become necessary. The editors/author/contributors have, as far as it is possible, taken care to ensure that the information given in this book is accurate and up-to-date. In view of the possibility of human error or advances in medical science neither the author nor the publisher nor any other party who has been involved in the preparation or publication of this work warrants that the information contained herein is in every respect accurate or complete. Readers are strongly advised to confirm.

Printed in USA

Dedicated to

Prof. Rais-ur-Rahman

for his constant encouragement and support

"Victory lies in every step, not at the end of the race alone"

Preface

Quite frequently these days people talk of Diabetes Mellitus as global problem, disease has been described in Unani System of Medicine in detail by the name Ziabetus Shakri. This book is aimed to provide concise introduction of the disease along with specific mention to basic approaches in a diabetes patient. It is hoped that this book shall provide evidence based guidelines about Diabetes to all readers.

I am highly indebted to my friends and colleagues for providing the necessary stimulus for writing this book. I am grateful to all those persons whose writings and works have helped me in the preparation of this book. I am equally grateful to the reviewer of the manuscript of this book who made extremely valuable suggestions and has thus contributed in enhancing the standard of the book. I shall feel amply rewarded if the book proves helpful to the diabetics. I look forward to suggestions from all readers for further improving the subject content as well as the presentation of this book.

Adnan Mastan

Contents

INTRODUCTION

Diabetes is a major public health problem and considered as one of the most common non-communicable disease, globally. Although the prevalence rate of the disease varies country to country. However, WHO has projected India as the country with the fastest growing population of diabetes patients. Due to its consequences Diabetes has become a silent killer that kills one person every 10 seconds, and worldwide it kills 3.2 millions every year. In Unani System of Medicine Diabetes is known by the name Ziabetus. Unani physician have been treating diabetes since ancient times; they have described a number of Unani drugs both single and compound for the management of Diabetes.

The term Ziabetus is a Greek word which means "to run through" or "Siphon", is characterized by hyperglycaemia, glycosuria, increased appetite, excessive thirst and gradual loss of body weight. Dayasqoomas, Qaramees, Dawwara, Dolab, Zalaq-ul-kuliya, Salesul-baul, Istisqae anmas, Barkarya, Moattasa and Attasa are the synonyms commonly used for Ziabetus in Unani System of Medicine. In Ziabetus, the patient excretes water as such through urinary passage soon after its intake. The ratio of fluid taken and the urinary output remains the same (Zalqul Majari) as that of solid without digestion from the stomach and intestine, a condition in Unani medicine as 'Zalqul-ama'. There is excessive thirst more intake of water and its rapid discharge as urine. The patient also experiences a feeling of heat in the back around the waist and in the right side of the body. When the disease takes the body completely in its grip dryness will develop all over the body rendering it weak.

There are four major causes described in most of the classical Unani literature, responsible for the development of Ziabetus:

1

1. Sue Mizaj har kulliya (Abnormal hot temperament of kidney).

2. Zoufe-kuliya (Weakness of kidney).

3. Majari ka kushada ho jana (Dilatation of renal vessels).

4. Sue mizaj barid of tamam badan / kuliya / jigar (Abnormal cold temperament of body / kidney / liver).

Among all above mentioned causes, most emphasis was given to abnormal hot temperament of kidney by most of the eminent Unani physicians during the description of Ziabetus. They also described that weakness of kidney and dilatation of renal vessels occurs due to abnormal hot temperament of kidney.

Ziabetus Can Be Divided Into Two Types:

(A) Ziabetus har and (B) Ziabetus barid

(A) Ziabetus bar: In this disease the patient feels very much thirst and passes white coloured urine frequently and the urine contains sugar. In fact it is the Diabetes in true sense. The excretion of sugar renders the body weak, the muscles degenerated and become lean and thin and the general health is run down.

B) Ziabetus barid: In this condition the patient feels acute thirst and passes white coloured urine in large quantity but does not contain sugar. This type of Ziabetus can be matched with Diabetes Insipidus.

In Modern system of Medicine Diabetes is when blood glucose*, also called blood sugar, is too high. Blood glucose is the main type of sugar found in blood and main source of energy. Glucose comes from the food we eat and is also made in our liver and muscles. Our blood carries glucose to all our body's cells to use for energy.

Our pancreas—an organ, located between stomach and spine, that helps with digestion—releases a hormone it makes, called insulin, into our blood. Insulin helps our blood carry glucose to all our body's cells. Sometimes our body doesn't make enough insulin or the insulin doesn't work the way it should. Glucose then stays in our blood and doesn't reach cells. As a result blood glucose levels get too high and can cause diabetes or prediabetes.

Over time, having too much glucose in our blood can cause health problems.

What is prediabetes?

Prediabetes is when the amount of glucose in our blood is above normal yet not high enough to be called diabetes. With prediabetes, chances of getting type 2 diabetes, heart disease, and stroke are higher. With some weight loss and moderate physical activity, we can delay or prevent type 2 diabetes. We can even return to normal glucose levels, possibly without taking any medicines.

Nowadays the accepted concept of Diabetes mellitus is that, it is a chronic disease of carbohydrate metabolism and glucose intolerance, characterized by high blood glucose level and glycosuria resulting from dysfunction of pancreatic β cells and insulin resistance. The defective β cells result in lack of total or partial synthesis of Insulin. Chronic hyperglycaemia also affects metabolism of protein and lipids.

HISTORY

Ziabetus is known since the age of antiquity, where symptoms of Ziabetus were described. It is commonly believed that the history of medicine began with the Greeks, and before the time of **Buqrat (460 BC)**, Ancient Egypt (Misri) was the first civilization known to have an extensive study of medicine and to have left behind written records of its practices and procedures. It is proved by the discovery of the **Ebers papyrus** in the graves of thabes by famous German Egyptologist **Georg Ebers** in 1862 AD. The Ebers papyrus is one of the most famous document relating to the ancient practice of medicine, written about 1550 BC. Ebers papyrus contains descriptions of various diseases including polyuric state resembling Ziabetus shakri. Although the Unani physician **Buqrat (460 BC)** "The father of medicine" did not specifically mentioned Ziabetus in his Writings, there are accounts in the Buqrat's writings that are consistent with the sign and symptoms of Ziabetus, like excessive urinary flow with wasting of the body. **Arsyatoos (Aretaeus)** and **Jalinoos (Galen)** were followers of Buqrat. **Arsyatoos (81-138 AD)** provided the first accurate description of the symptoms of Ziabetus. He was the first who use the term **"Ziabetus"** in connection with this ailment, which means "to run trough" or "Siphon". He described the disease as "Ziabetus is a dreadful affliction, not very frequently among men, being a melting down of the flesh and limbs into urine". **Jalinoos (131-201 AD),** a contemporary of Arsyatoos, the most influential medical writer of all time, discussed Ziabetus in a number of his books. He described the condition as rare, as he had only seen two cases; he referred to the ailment as "Diarrhoea Urinosa (Diarrhoea of urine)" and "dipsakos (the thirsty disease)". However, the association of polyuric with a sweet tasting substance in the urine was first reported in Sanskrit literature dating from the 5th - 6th century AD at the time of **Susruta, Charaka and Vaghbata**. They described the urine of polyuric patients as having the taste like honey, being sticky to touch and strongly attracting the ants. The Indian description of that time also contains Ziabetus like conditions of two types: Congenital and late onset. Also, the Indians noticed the relation of Ziabetus to heredity, obesity, sedentary life and diet. During the same era, Chinese and Japanese physicians also described Ziabetus and the sweetness of urine of Ziabetus patients, which apparently attracted dogs. They also observed that people with Ziabetus were prone to develop boils and an affliction which clinically resembles tuberculosis. During the 9th - 11th AD, Arabic medicine was at its peak of achievements and Arabian physicians translated the works of Buqrat and Jalinoos and enriched them with latest knowledge of that era. Two prominent physicians of this era who contributed to the knowledge of were **Shaikh-Ul-Rais Bu Ali Ibne Sina (960-1037 AD)** and **Musa Bin Maimoon (1135 AD).** Ibne Sina described accurately the clinical features of the disease and mentioned two specific complications of the disease, namely gangrene and the collapse of sexual function. While on the other hand Musa Bin Maimoon claimed to have seen more than 20 cases. He proposed that Ziabetus was caused by the sweet water of river Nile and the prevailing heat that spreads over the kidneys. No further progress was made in the understanding of Ziabetus until the 16th century AD. When the Swiss physician **Von Hohenheim (Paracelsus)** reported that urine of Ziabetus (Diabetic): Patients contained an abnormal substance which remained as a white powder after evaporation; he concluded that this substance was salt and that Diabetes was due to the deposition of salt in the kidneys causing thirst of the kidney and polyuria. The modern history of Diabetes began with the **Thomas Willi's (1621-1675 AD)** observations of Diabetes in 1674 AD and **Matthew Dobson's** experiments in 1776 AD that conclusively established the diagnosis of Diabetes in the presence of sugar in the urine and blood. Diabetes was no longer considered a rare ailment. Thomas Willis referred to Diabetes as the "Pissing evil" and noted that in patients with Diabetes, "The urine was

5

wonderfully sweet, as if it were imbued with honey or sugar". He claimed that Diabetes was primarily a disease of the blood and not the kidneys. Willis proposed that the sweetness first appeared in the blood and was later found in the urine. During the same era **Thomas Sydenham (1624-1689 AD)** speculated that Diabetes was a systemic disease arising in the blood where "Chyle" was incompletely digested and its non-absorbed residue had to be excreted. After Thomas Sydenham, **Johann Conrada Brunner (1653-1727 AD)** came very close to discovering pancreatic Diabetes when he observed in 1682 AD that, After the incomplete removal of the pancreas from a dog,

"…... the animal made water very frequently and that he was very thirsty, drinking largely water in proportion to the discharge of urine". **Cullen** was the person who distinguished Diabetes into two types. In this classification, we find first time a distinction between Diabetes, with the urine of "the smell; colour and flavor of honey," and Diabetes, with limpid but not sweet urine. The concept of Thomas was further elaborated by **Matthew Dobson (1735-1784 AD),** who provided experimental evidence that people with Diabetes pass sugar in their urine. He gently heated two quarts of urine to dryness. The remaining residue was a whitish cake, which Dobson wrote " was granulated and broke easily between the fingers; it smelled sweet like brown sugar, neither could it be distinguished from sugar, except that the sweetness left a slight sense of coolness on the palate". Moreover he concluded that this substance had previously existed in the serum rather than being formed in the kidneys. He wrote "this idea of the disease explains its emaciating effects from so large a proportion of the alimentary matter being drawn off by the kidneys, before it is perfectly assimilated and applied to the purpose of nutrition. In 1788 AD **Thomas Cawley** described that; Diabetes may follow damage to the pancreas, such as through calculus formation. Twenty years after the Matthew Dobson, in 1797 AD **Matthew Baillie** stated that "upon examination of the kidneys...... it seemed probable that Diabetes depends, in a considerable degree, upon a deranged action of the secretory structure of the kidneys, by which the blood there is disposed to new combinations" the effect of which is the production of "a saccharine matter". He also proposed that "the chyle may be so imperfectly formed, as to make the blood be more readily changed into a saccharine matter by the action of the kidneys". In 1798 AD, a year after the Matthew Baillie, "**John Rollo**" a surgeon, expressed his opinion that "the Diabetes Mellitus" is a disease of the stomach and its immediate cause is a morbid condition of stomach evolving from vegetable substances containing saccharine matter, which is quickly separated as a foreign body by the kidney". Further he was the first who use the adjective "Mellitus" to distinguish the condition from other polyuric diseases in which glycosuria was absent and urine was tasteless. Rollo made other contributions to the study of Diabetes, including descriptions of "cataract due to Diabetes" and odour of acetone on the breath of some Diabetes patients. In 1815 AD, **Michel Eugene Chevreul (1786-1889 AD)** published his experimental findings on urine and stated that sweet substance found in urine of Diabetes patients was to be identical to grape sugar. In 1839 AD, **John Elliston** speaks about "grief', "chills" and, "excess of venery" as possible etiological factors for Diabetes in his "Principles and practice of medicine". In the first half of the 19th century **Claude Bernard (1813-1878 AD)** discovered that the liver releases a substance that affects blood sugar levels. In 1875 AD, he isolated a starch like substance that he called "Glycogen", which was the precursor of glucose, "the internal secretion" of the liver. This observation established the liver's role as a vital organ in Diabetes. He also demonstrated that the central nervous system was involved in controlling the blood glucose concentration. He also performed many systematic experiments on the pancreas. During mid 19th century AD, **William Prout (1785-1859 AD)** described "exposure to cold", "attacks of rheumatism and gout", "The drinking of cold fluids while heated and "mental anxiety and distress" as the most frequent exciting causes of Diabetes. He was the first, who recognized the coma as a complication of Diabetes. Further in 1869 AD, **H.D.Noyes**, observed that a form of "retinitis" developed in glycosuric patients, during the same year, **Paul Langrhans (1847-1888 AD)** had noticed small clusters of ductless cells in teased preparations of pancreas, he simply described these structures without speculating as to their possible function. It was only in 1893 AD that **Edouard Laguesse (1861-1927 AD)** suggested that these clumps of cells, which he named the **"islets of langerhans"** in honour of langerhans and suggested that they might constitute the endocrine tissue of the pancreas. In 1874 AD, **Prof.A.Kussmaul (1822-1902 AD)** described the "air hunger" of ketoacidosis. In1875 AD, **Dickinson** published a paper "Diabetes, in his diseases of the kidneys", in which he defined Diabetes as "a disease of the nervous system characterized by the secretion of saccharine containing urine". In 1877 AD, **Etienne Lancereaux (1829-910 AD)** demonstrated a causal relationship between Diabetes and lesions of the pancreas and his friend, **Apollinaire Bauchardat (1806-1886 AD),** began the modern therapy of Diabetes by limiting carbohydrates in the diet, advocating fast days and using exercise to help control glycosuria. In 1889 AD, **Oskar Minkowski (1858-1931 AD)** and **Josef Von Mering (1849-1908 AD)** demonstrated conclusively that removal of the pancreas from a dog results in the development of fatal Diabetes. This observation firmly established the role of the pancreatic disorders in causing Diabetes. Further in 1901 AD, **Eugene Undsay Opie's (1873-1962 AD)** pathologic study on Diabetes Mellitus established that Diabetes is caused by a lesion of the pancreas and the lesion is of such kind in which the islands of langerhans are destroyed or injured. In1908 AD, **Georg L.Zuelzer (1870-1949 AD)** and **Nicolas Paulesco (1869-1931AD)** had prepared potent pancreatic extract before 1921 AD. In 1909 AD, **Jean De Meyer**

8

gave the name "insulin" derived from the latin word insula (insula=island), to the glucose lowering hormone, whose existence at that time was still hypothetical, which he postulated was produced by the islet tissue. Further **Moses Barron (1883 AD)** give conclusion regarding the relationship of islets of langerhans to Diabetes ".......that the islets secrete a hormone directly into the lymph or blood streams (Internal secretion), which has a controlling power over carbohydrate metabolism". The finding of Moses Barron triggered the investigations of **Frederick Grant Banting (1891-1941 AD)** and **Charles Herbert Best (1899 AD)**. In December 1921 AD, they got success in isolation of insulin and published the results of their research on "The internal secretion of the pancreas" in which they were able to demonstrate the reversal of the metabolic changes of Diabetes by injection of a potent extract of the pancreatic islands. On 11th Jan 1922 AD, the first patient of Diabetes a 14 year old boy named **Leonard Thombson** was treated with insulin. In 1923 AD Eli Lilly begins commercial production of insulin, and called it "Isletin Insulin." In 1925 AD Home testing for sugar in the urine through Benedict's solution was introduced. In 1927 AD an oral medication called "horment" or "glukohorment" was developed as a replacement for insulin, but side effects are unacceptable and very soon dropped out. In 1930s AD Insulin as further refined to Protamine zinc insulin, a long-acting insulin that provide more flexibility. In 1936 AD **Himsworth** divided Diabetics into two types based on "insulin sensitivity." In 1940's AD neutral protamine Hagedorn insulin was introduced and the connection was established between Diabetes and long-term complications of kidney and eye diseases. In late 1940's AD **Helen Free** developed the "dip-and-read" urine test (Clinistix) allowing instant monitoring of blood glucose levels. In 1951 AD **Lawrence Bornstein** measured the amount of insulin in the blood and noted that older and obese patients with Diabetes have insulin, but those who were young have none. In 1955 AD Oral drugs that help lower blood glucose levels was introduced. In 1959 AD, Two major types of diabetes are recognized: Type 1 (Insulin-Dependent) Diabetes and Type 2 (Non-Insulin-Dependent) Diabetes. During the 1959-1960 AD **Yallow** and **Berson** developed the radioimmunological assay (RIA) procedure, to measure insulin with much greater precision than earlier techniques, for that Yallow received the Nobel Prize in 1977 AD. In 1964 AD, The first strips for testing blood glucose were used. In1970 AD, First blood glucose meter (Ames) and Insulin pumps were introduced. During the same year Laser therapy was used to slow down or prevent blindness due to Diabetes. In1973 AD, U-100 insulin is introduced. In 1976 AD, the glycosylated haemoglobin (HbAlC) test was introduced as a monitor of glycaemic control. The manufacturing of insulin changed dramatically with the advent of DNA technology that allows synthesis of a genetically engineered "human" type of insulin, and in 1978 AD, production of the first recombinant DNA insulin was announced. In 1979 AD, Type 1 and Type 2 Diabetes are formally recognized by the American Diabetes Association. Type 1 is also called Insulin Dependent Diabetes Mellitus (IDDM), and Type 2 is called Non Insulin Dependent Diabetes Mellitus (NIDDM). In 1983 AD, the first biosynthetic human insulin, and "Reflolux", later known as "Accu-Chek"(allows blood glucose self-monitoring) was introduced. In 1996 AD, the FDA approved the first recombinant DNA human insulin analogue, lispro (Humalog). In 2001 AD, FDA approved Cygnus' first-generation model of the GlucoWatch Biographer for use by adults - the first frequent, automatic and non-invasive glucose monitor. In 2003 AD, the names Insulin Dependent Diabetes Mellitus (IDDM) for Type 1 and Non Insulin Dependent Diabetes Mellitus (NIDDM) for Type 2 diabetes are formally dropped. Today Researchers are working on an insulin patch and inhaled insulin, Genetic engineering is being used to manipulate cells so they secrete insulin. A sensor-computer-pump system that mimics the insulin response of the normal pancreas is being developed to function as an "artificial pancreas". Apart from these, various researches are still going on, to explore new aspects of Diabetes and its management.

PREVALENCE

Diabetes is now one of the most common non-communicable diseases globally. It is a silent killer that kills one person every 10 seconds, and worldwide it kills about 3.2   million every year. At least one in ten deaths among adults between 35-64 years old is attributable to Diabetic. Further it is the fourth or fifth leading cause of death in most developed countries and there is substantial evidence that it is epidemic in many and newly industrialized nations. Diabetes Mellitus is certain to be one of the most challenging health problems in the 21st century. Type 2 Diabetes Mellitus constitutes about   85 to   95% of all Diabetes in developed countries and accounts for an even higher percentage in developing countries. Type   2 Diabetes Mellitus is now a common and serious global health problem, which, for most countries has evolved in association with rapid cultural and social changes, ageing populations, increasing urbanization, dietary changes, reduced physical activity and other lifestyle and behavioral patterns.

The number of people around the world suffering from the diabetes has skyrocketed in last two decades, from 20 to 250 million. South East Asian countries have the highest burden of diabetes. Major contribution to diabetic population in Southeast Asia is from India. It has been estimated that India, considered as the diabetic capital of the world with more than 40 million diabetes patients, would continue to lead even at 2030 with a whopping 80 million diabetics.

Table 1. Expected Diabetes status in 2015

All Diabetes	2025
Total world population in billions	7.9
Adult population in billions (20-79 years)	5.2
Number of people with diabetes in millions	380
World diabetes prevalence %	7.3
Number of people with diabetes in India in millions	69.9

Age Distribution

The 40-59 year age group currently has the highest number of persons of Diabetes with some 113 million (46 % of total world Diabetic population), of which more than 70 % live in developing countries.

Gender Distribution

The estimates for both 2003 and 2025 showed a female predominance in the number of persons with diabetes. The female numbers were about 10% higher than for males.

Urban/Rural Distribution

In 2003, the number of people with diabetes in urban areas was 78 million, compared to 44 million persons with diabetes in rural areas. By 2025, it is expected that this discrepancy will increase to 182 million urban and 61 million rural persons with diabetes. In India prevalence of diabetes in urban population is 5.9 % and in rural population it is 2.7%.

CLASSIFICATION

In Unani system of Medicine Ziabetus Can Be Divided Into Two Types:

(A) Ziabetus har and (B) Ziabetus barid

(A) Ziabetus bar: In this disease the patient feels very much thirst and passes white coloured urine frequently and the urine contains sugar. In fact it is the Diabetes in true sense. The excretion of sugar renders the body weak, the muscles degenerated and become lean and thin and the general health is run down.

B) Ziabetus barid: In this condition the patient feels acute thirst and passes white coloured urine in large quantity but does not contain sugar. This type of Ziabetus can be matched with Diabetes Insipidus.

As per Modern concept there are three main types of diabetes are type 1, type 2, and gestational diabetes. People can develop diabetes at any age. Both women and men can develop diabetes.

Type 1 Diabetes

Type 1 diabetes, which used to be called juvenile diabetes, develops most often in young people; however, type 1 diabetes can also develop in adults. In type 1 diabetes, your body no longer makes insulin or enough insulin because the body's immune system, which normally protects you from infection by getting rid of bacteria, viruses, and other harmful substances, has attacked and destroyed the cells that make insulin.

Type 2 Diabetes

Type 2 diabetes, which used to be called adult-onset diabetes, can affect people at any age, even children. However, type 2 diabetes develops most often in middle-aged and older people. People who are overweight and inactive are also more likely to develop type 2 diabetes.

Type 2 diabetes usually begins with insulin resistance—a condition that occurs when fat, muscle, and liver cells do not use insulin to carry glucose into the body's cells to use for energy. As a result, the body needs more insulin to help glucose enter cells. At first, the pancreas keeps up with the added demand by making more insulin. Over time, the pancreas doesn't make enough insulin when blood sugar levels increase, such as after meals. If your pancreas can no longer make enough insulin, you will need to treat your type 2 Diabetes.

Gestational Diabetes

Gestational diabetes can develop when a woman is pregnant. Pregnant women make hormones that can lead to insulin resistance. All women have insulin resistance late in their pregnancy. If the pancreas doesn't make enough insulin during pregnancy, a woman develops gestational diabetes.

Overweight or obese women have a higher chance of gestational diabetes. Also, gaining too much weight during pregnancy may increase your likelihood of developing gestational diabetes.

Gestational diabetes most often goes away after the baby is born. However, a woman who has had gestational diabetes is more likely to develop type 2 diabetes later in life. Babies born to mothers who had gestational diabetes are also more likely to develop obesity and type 2 diabetes.

Other specific types

   A. Genetic Defects Of Cell Function

- Chromosome 12, HNF-1(MODY3)

- Chromosome 7, glucokinase (MODY2)

- Chromosome 20, HNF-4 (MODY1)

- Chromosome 13, insulin promoter factor-1(IPF-1; MODY4)

- Chromosome 17, HNF-1 (MODY5)

- Chromosome 2, NeuroDI (MODY6)

- Mitochondria DNA

- Others

B. Genetic Defects of insulin Action

- **Type A** insulin resistance

- Leprechaunism

- Rabson-Mendenhall syndrome

- Lipoatrophic Diabetes

- Others

C. Diseases of the Exocrine Pancreas

- Pancreatitis

- Trauma/pancreatectomy

- Neoplasia

- Cystic fibrosis

- Heamochromatosis

- Fibrocalculous pancreatopathy

- Others

D. Endocrinopathies

- Acromegaly

- Cushing's syndrome

- Glucagonoma

- Pheochromocytoma

- Somatostatinoma

- Aldosteronoma

- Others

E. Drug or Chemical-Induced

- Vacor

- Pentamidine

- Nicotinic acid

- Glucocorticoids

- Thyroid hormone

- Diazoxide

- Adrenergic agonists

- Thiazides

- Dilantin

- Interferon

- Others

F. Infections

- Congenital rubella

- Cytomegalovirus

- Others

G. Uncommon forms of Immune-Mediated Diabetes

- "Stiff-man" Syndrome

- Anti—insulin receptor antibodies

- Others

H. Other Genetic Syndromes Sometimes Associated With Diabetes

- Down's Syndrome

- Klinefelter's syndrome

- Turner's syndrome

- Wolfram's

- Friedreich's ataxia

- Huntington's chorea

- Laurence-Moon-Biedl

- Myotonic dystrophy

- Porphyria

- Prader-Willi syndrome

- Others

PATHOGENESIS

Pathogenesis of Ziabetus Shakri (Diabetes Mellitus) In Unani System of Medicine

In Unani system of medicine, ancient Philosophers explained the pathogenesis of Shakri (Diabetes Mellitus) logically and rationally. The mainstay of Ziabetus is the development of abnormal hot temperament in the kidney. This altered hot temperament renders the renal vessels paralyzed and hence dilated. The morbid hot temperament disturbs the normal functioning of kidney and reduces the Quwwate Masika (Retentive power) of kidney. In contrast to the reduced retentive power, the morbid hot temperament, on the other hand increases the Quwwate Jazba (Absorptive power) of The excessive thrust of Quwwate Jazba pulls and absorbs the excessively large amount of water from the liver but as unable to digest and retain the fluid due to weak Quwwate fasika and strengthen Quwwate Dafia, the fluid ultimately passes out towards bladder and finally in the form of urine large amount of fluid excreted. The deficit of fluid thus created in the liver is compensated by excessive absorption of fluid from the Urooqe Masariqa (Mesenteric vessels). The Urooqe Masariqa absorbs the fluid from the stomach, and stomach demands plentiful fluid from outside in form of excessive thirst. The concentration of this demand and supply thus established between the organs, vicious cycle resulting in large intake of fluid as due to thirst and thereof and frequent urination.

Pathogenesis of Diabetes Mellitus Type 2 In Modern System of Medicine

Type 2 Diabetes Mellitus known as maturity onset type of Diabetes till 1979 AD and non insulin dependent Diabetes thereafter, it accounts for 85 to 95 % of all patients with Diabetes mellitus. Pathogenesis of this primary form of Diabetes Mellitus is complex and varied. The disorder evolves slowly in course of several years with a clinical phase. Two distinct factors that work in tandem for the evolution and progress of the disorder are:

A. Insulin secretory dysfunction i.e. failure of pancreatic β cells to release as much insulin as required for metabolic control under the prevailing situation "relative insulin deficiency".

B. Impaired insulin action manifest as decreased insulin sensitivity of the target cells "insulin resistance".

Both insulin secretory function and sensitivity to insulin action are modulated by hereditary and environmental factors.

1. **Insulin Secretory Dysfunction:** Impaired insulin secretion is a uniform finding in Diabetic patients and the development of beta cell dysfunction has been well characterized in diverse ethnic populations. Early in the natural history of type-2 Diabetes Mellitus, insulin resistance with loss or reduction of 1st phase and prolongation of 2nd phase of insulin secretion is well established, but glucose tolerance remains normal because of a compensatory increase in insulin secretion. Within the normal glucose tolerant population, approximately 20-25 % of individuals are severely resistant to the action of insulin. However, insulin secretion in these insulin resistant Non-Diabetic Individuals is increased in proportion to the severity of insulin resistance and glucose tolerance remains normal. As the fasting plasma glucose concentration rises from 80 to 140 mg/dl, the fasting plasma insulin concentration increases progressively, up to two to three fold above that in normal glucose tolerant subjects. The progressive rise in fasting plasma insulin level is an adaptive response of the pancreas to maintain normal glucose homeostasis. However, when the fasting plasma glucose concentration rises above 140

mg/dl, it causes glucotoxicity to β cells and affects insulin gene transcription, leading to decreased insulin synthesis and secretion. Hyperglycaemia and hypoinsulinaemia causes lipotoxicity to β cells by increasing plasma free fatty acid (FFA) levels which make situation worse, because prolonged exposure of β cells to elevated plasma FFA levels leads to further inhibition of insulin secretion. Increased fatty acyl CoA levels within the 13 cells also impair beta cell function and causes apoptosis of beta cells   . Apart from gluco-lipotoxicity, some other factors contribute to beta cell dysfunction and leads to impaired insulin secretion like Incretin deficiency and / or incretin resistance and hyper secretion of amylin. Apart from these acquired causes some genetic factors are also implicated in inducing defect in β cell function. Monogenic mutations leading to defects in insulin secretion have been documented in five types of maturity onset type of Diabetes in the young (MODY) and two clusters with mitochondrial DNA mutation thus for such patients may account for 1 % of Non-insulin dependent Diabetes among the Caucasians Specification of genetic loci in the rest still continues to remain as nightmare for geneticists.

2. **Impaired Insulin Action Or Insulin Resistance:**   Insulin resistance implies decreased peripheral uptake of glucose as well as inadequate suppression of hepatic glucose production and lipolysis in response to insulin. Relatively high levels of insulin at fasting and in response to secretogogues are indicative of insulin resistance. Insulin resistance is well known in obesity, because obesity is an extremely important diabetogenic influence and not surprisingly, approximately 80 % of Type-2 Diabetes Mellitus patients are obese.

Seats of Insulin Resistance

A. **Muscle:** Skeletal muscles and adipose tissues required insulin for optimal glucose uptake and utilization. In Type-2 Diabetes Mellitus, entry of glucose into myocytes occurs only through mass action as available insulin fails to recruit more GLUT 4 for facilitated transport of glucose across the cell membrane, and result in reduction of glucose uptake. Further insulin mediated augmentation of glucose utilization is impaired in muscles of patients with Type-2 Diabetes Mellitus. Late increase in the contents of triglycerides in skeletal muscles has been implicated to induce insulin resistance in the muscles.

B. **Liver:** In Type-2 Diabetes Mellitus restraining effects of insulin in hepatic glucose production (HGP) is impaired and leads to increase HGP during post absorptive and fasting states.

C. **Adipose Tissue:** Free fatty acids are stored as triglycerides in adipocytes and serve as an important energy source during conditions of fasting. Insulin is a potent inhibitor of lipolysis and restrains the release of FFA from the adipocytes by inhibiting the enzyme hormone sensitive lipase. In Type-2 Diabetics the ability of insulin to inhibit lipolysis and reduce the plasma FFA concentration is markedly reduced. Prolonged elevation of plasma FFA concentration leads to insulin resistance in muscles and liver thus impair insulin secretion.

Cellular Mechanism of Insulin Resistance: The stimulation of glucose metabolism by insulin requires that the hormone must first bind to specific receptors that are present on the cell surface of all insulin target tissues. After insulin has bound to and activated itsreceptors "second messengers" are generated which initiate a series of events that eventually result in the stimulation of intracellular glucose metabolism under the control of insulin. In Type-2 Diabetes Mellitus insulin binding to target tissue is reduced due to decreased number of receptors without change in insulin receptor affinity. In addition to the decreased number of cell surface receptors, a variety of defects in insulin receptor internalization and processing also occurred.

CLINICAL FEATURES

Certain risk factors make people more likely to develop type 2 diabetes. Some of these are

- A family history of diabetes.
- Lack of exercise.
- Weighing too much.
- Being of African American, American Indian, Alaska Native, Hispanic/Latino, or Asian/Pacific Islander heritage.
- Gestational diabetes history.

In classical Unani literature it is described that, the disease Ziabetus always clinically presents itself by:

1. Increased frequency of Micturition with excessive thirst and dryness of mouth.
2. Ants and flies are attracted on urine (Due to presence sugar).
3. Patients feel heat in the back around the waist (In case of abnormal hot temperament of kidney).
4. Dryness all over the body (Due to shortage of fluid in body).

While according to modern system of medicine, Type 2 Diabetes Mellitus develops slowly. Many people have Type 2 Diabetes for several years before the condition is diagnosed, often through routine screening tests. Typically, the earliest symptoms are increased thirst and frequent urination. That's because excess glucose circulating in body draws water from tissues, making patients dehydrated. To quench thirst, patients drink more water and other beverages which lead to more frequent urination.

The signs and symptoms of diabetes are

- being very thirsty

- urinating often

- feeling very hungry

- feeling very tired

- losing weight without trying

- sores that heal slowly

- dry, itchy skin

- feelings of pins and needles in your feet

- losing feeling in your feet

- blurry eyesight

Some people with diabetes don't have any of these signs or symptoms. The only way to know if you have diabetes is to have your doctor do a blood test.

COMPLICATIONS

In Diabetes as the vicious cycle of large intake of fluid and frequent urination developed, it affects almost all body parts. First, it weakened the liver due to which there is deficiency of fluid and nutrition to all body parts which initially results in generalized weakness, but with the passage of time it results in development of generalized wasting and dryness all over the body.

According To Modern Literature Complications Of Diabetes Mellitus Can Be Divided Into Two Types:

- ➢ Acute complications
- ➢ Chronic complications

Acute complications

- A. Diabetic ketoacidosis
- B. Nonketotic hyperosmolar coma
- C. Hypoglycemia
- D. Amputation

Chronic complications

- A. Microvascular diseases
- a. Diabetic retinopathy
    - ➢ Severe vision loss
    - ➢ Blindness.
- b. Diabetic neuropathy
    - ➢ Abnormal sensation

> ➢ Decreased sensation

> ➢ Diabetic foot

c. Diabetic nephropathy- chronic renal failure

B. Macrovascular disease

a. Atherosclerosis

b. Coronary artery disease, leading to myocardial infarction or angina

c. Stroke (mainly ischemic type)

d. Peripheral vascular disease, which contributes to intermittent claudication (exertion-related foot pain) as well as diabetic foot

e. Diabetic myonecrosis

f. Diabetic foot often due to a combination of neuropathy and arterial disease.

DIAGNOSTIC CRITERIA

Checking and recording your blood glucose levels can help you monitor and better manage your diabetes. If your blood has too much or too little glucose, you may need a change in your healthy eating plan, physical activity plan, or medicines.

You may need to check before and after eating, before and after physical activity, before bed, and sometimes in the middle of the night. Make sure to keep a record of your blood glucose self-checks.

Revised criteria for diagnosing Diabetes Mellitus (Ziabetus Shakri) have been issued by consensus panel of experts from the National Diabetes data group and the world health organization. The revised criteria reflect new epidemiologic and metabolic evidence and are based on the following premises:

1. The spectrum of fasting plasma glucose and the response to an oral glucose load varies in normal individuals.

2. Diabetes Mellitus defined as the level of glycaemia at which Diabetes specific complications are noted and not on the level of glucose tolerance from population based viewpoint.

In the new diagnostic criteria the oral glucose tolerance test which was previously recommended by the National Diabetes Data group has been replaced with the recommendation that the diagnosis of Diabetes Mellitus be based on:

➤ Two consecutive readings of fasting plasma glucose levels of 126 mg/dl (7.0 mmol/L) or higher.

Other options for diagnosis include:

➢ Two consecutive readings of casual plasma glucose concentration (Random) 200 mg /dl (11.1 mmol / L) or higher with symptoms of Diabetes i.e. polyuria, polydipsia or unexplained weight loss. Casual is defined as any time of day without regard to time since last meal.

Or

➢ Finding of two consecutive readings of two hour post prandial plasma glucose readings ≥200 mg /dl during an oral glucose tolerance test.

Fasting plasma glucose is selected as the primary diagnostic test because it predicts adverse outcomes (e.g. retinopathy) as well as the two hour post prandial blood glucose test. But fasting plasma glucose is much more reproducible than oral glucose tolerance test or the Random blood glucose test and easier to perform in a clinical setting.

Criteria for Testing For Diabetes Mellitus In Asymptomatic Undiagnosed Individuals:

1. Testing for Diabetes should be considered in all individuals at age 45 years and above and, if normal, it should be repeated at 3 years intervals.

2. Testing should be considered at a young age or be carried out more frequently in individuals who are

➢ Obese (> 120% desirable body weight or a BMI > 27 kg /m2)

➢ Habitually physically inactive

➢ Have a first degree relative with Diabetes

➢ Members of a high risk ethnic population

- Have delivered a baby weighing >9 lb (i.e.> 4.032 kg) or Have been diagnosed with Gestational Diabetes Mellitus

- Hypertensive (BP > 140/90 mm Hg)

- Have a HDL cholesterol level < 35 mg /dl (0.90 mmol /L) and / or a triglyceride level > 250 mg /dl (2.82 mmol/L)

- On previous testing, had Impaired Glucose Tolerance or Impaired Fasting Glucose

The A1C Test

Another test for blood glucose, the A1C—also called the hemoglobin A1C test, HbA1C, or glycohemoglobin test—is a blood test that reflects the average level of glucose in your blood during the past 2 to 3 months.

You should have the A1C test at least twice a year. If your result is not on target, your doctor may have you take the test more often to see if your A1C improves.

For the test, doctor will draw a sample of blood during an office visit or send you to a lab to have your blood drawn. A1C test result is given as a percentage. Your A1C result plus the record of your blood glucose numbers show whether your blood glucose levels are under control.

If your A1C result is too high, you may need to change your diabetes treatment plan.

If your A1C result is on target, then your diabetes treatment plan is working. The lower your A1C result, the lower your chance of having diabetes problems.

Table 2. A1C Targets

A1C Targets	
Target for most people with diabetes	Below 7 percent
Time to change my diabetes care plan	8 percent or above

Tests for Ketones

You may need to check your blood or urine for ketones if you're sick or if your blood glucose levels are above 240. Your body makes ketones when you burn fat instead of glucose for energy. If you have too many ketones, you are more likely to have a serious condition called ketoacidosis. If not treated, ketoacidosis can cause death.

Signs of ketoacidosis are

- vomiting
- weakness
- fast breathing
- sweet-smelling breath

Ketoacidosis is more likely in people with type 1 diabetes.

MANAGEMENT OF DIABETES AND APPROACHES FOR A DIABETIC PATIENT

Studies show that keeping your blood glucose (also called blood sugar) close to normal helps prevent or delay some diabetes problems. Through careful control, many problems such as eye disease, kidney disease, heart disease, nerve damage, and serious foot problems can be prevented or slowed. People who have type 1diabetes as well as people who have type 2 diabetes can benefit by keeping their blood glucose levels closer to normal.

As the turtle makes steady progress, so too must those with diabetes continue to maintain healthy lifestyles and stick to daily routines that involve regular exercise, good nutrition, glucose monitoring, and regular visits to health care providers.

The goals of management in people with Ziabetus Shakri (Diabetes Mellitus) are:

➢ To normalize the elevated blood sugar level.

➢ Relief from Diabetic symptoms and improvement in quality of life.

➢ Prevention of acute complications.

➢ Prevention of microvascular complications like retinopathy, neuropathy and nephropathy.

➢ Prevention of macrovascular complications like cardiovascular, cerebrovascular and peripheral vascular disease.

➢ Prevention of infections.

To keep your glucose at a healthy level, you need to keep a balance between three important things:

➢ What you eat and drink.

> How much physical activity you do.

> What diabetes medicine you take (if your doctor has prescribed diabetes pills or insulin).

Nutritional Approach for Diabetic

There is renewed interest in the prevention of insulin resistance and type 2 diabetes through lifestyle interventions. The key lifestyle interventions are physical activity and a nutritional plan set up with reduced caloric intake. Nutrition and lifestyle education programmes have been shown to be effective in delaying the onset of Type 2 diabetes and in achieving treatment goals for intermediate risk factors like as glycaemia, lipids, and blood pressure. There is now strong evidence from randomized, controlled trials that lifestyle interventions incorporating diet and physical activity can prevent Type 2 diabetes in high risk individuals from different ethnic backgrounds and that intensive lifestyle interventions are rated as very cost-effective. The risk of Type 2 diabetes is reduced by 28 to 59 per cent after implementation of lifestyle change. The main components of these lifestyle interventions included weight loss, reduction in fat intake and increased physical activity. The most dominant predictor for Type 2 diabetes prevention is weight loss; every kilogram lost is associated with a 16 per cent reduction in risk. However, there is little evidence supporting the most effective approach for weight reduction in people at risk of Type 2 diabetes.

Table3. Dietary component and related Diabetes Risk

Dietary component	Factors related to reduced risk	Factors related to increased risk
Nutrients		
Carbohydrate: Glycaemic index		High GI diets increase risk by 40%. Highest quintile (mean GI = 83.1) associated with 59% increased risk
Wholegrains	Wholegrains have a protective effect. Highest quintile (mean 3.2 servings/day) associated with risk reduction of 31%	
Fat: Total and Saturated Fat	Replacing saturated fat with unsaturated fat has a beneficial effect on insulin sensitivity	
Protein: Red meat		Relative risk increased by 26% for each serving increase of red meat
Processed meat		Processed meat increases risk. Highest quintile (5servings/week) associated with 46% increased risk Relative risk increased by 19% for each serving increase of processed meat.
Specific foods: Dairy products	Dairy products are protective. Each serving/ day increase is associated with a risk reduction of 9 % in men and 4% in women	
Fruit and vegetables	Green leafy vegetables reduce risk, an increase of 1.15 servings/day associated with 14% decrease in incidence[28] highest quintile (median 1.42 servings/day) associated with risk reduction of ~30%	

Coffee	4 or more cups/day decreases risk by 47%	
Alcohol	58% risk reduction associated with 15 – 29.9g/ day (1.5 – 3 UK units)	
Potatoes and fried Potatoes		2 weekly servings of fried potatoes increases risk by 16%

The nutrition plan for diabetes is the nutrition regimen developed to meet physical, metabolic, and lifestyle requirements of an individual. For patients with type 2 diabetes, reduction of total energy intake and increase in physical activity consistent with the patient's physical capabilities should be counseled in order to scale back body fat, decrease insulin resistance, and improve glycaemic and lipid control.

Table4. Dietary Recommendation for Diabetes

Component	Recommendation	Avoid
Total Calorie Intake	Depend on physical activity nutritional status of individual. The caloric intake of a person with diabetes should be altered gradually, preferably not more than 500 Kcal per day	
Total Calorie Distribution		
Carbohydrate (55-60% of total calorie requirement)	Main source should be cereals, mixed coarse grains, whole pulses, salads and soybeans.	Avoid sugar, honey, jiggery and sweets. Restrict processed refined food like maida-based products.
Protein (10-15% of total calorie requirement)	Preferably from vegetable sources, low fat milk and milk products, fish and lean meat.	
Fat (20-25% of total calorie requirement)	Saturated fat < 7% of total calorie intake. Rest should be in form of MUFA and PUFA. Use oils containing linoleic acid such as ground nut, sesame, and cotton seed.	Trans-fatty acid. Dietary cholesterol should be minimal.
Fibers	Whole grains (ragi, jowhar, barley, oats etc.), whole pulses, soybean, green leafy vegetables and fenu-greek seeds. Whole fruits in moderation	
Fruits	Upto 6g/day	Very sweet fruit and fruit juices.
Common Salt	Should be limited	Restrict Pickles, chatni, and salty processed foods.
Artificial Sweeteners		Avoid during pregnancy and lactation.
Dietary modification in Special situations		
Nephropathy	Protein should be restricted to 0.6 g/kg, and salt to 4 g/day.	
Hypertension	Dietary salt should be restricted to minimum.	
Dyslipidemia	Total fat intake should be curtailed and diet to be modified by increasing MUFA and dietary fiber.	Reducing saturated fatty acid.
Infections and acute illness	Adequate calorie must be ensured.	Avoid fasting

Dietary advice is no longer a list of instructions dictating what people with diabetes should or should not eat but to determine how current-eating habits can best be modified in order to meet the clinical objectives. Dietary change is achieved by a series of small stepwise changes rather than a major disruption. The extent and pace of change is thus a balance between what is desirable and what is acceptable. Dietary education is an ongoing interactive method of follow up, adjustment and support not a simply standard package delivered in a single session. Additional factors like individual circumstances, and cultural and ethnic preferences should be considered and the person with diabetes should also be involved in the decision making process. Dietary recommendations for the management of diabetes should focus more on the quality and quantity of carbohydrates and fat within the diet in addition to balancing total energy intake with expenditure. Thus, with a balanced diet with optimum nutrition, the diabetic individuals need no additional supplements for vitamins and minerals. Appropriate nutrition measures will help in reducing the risk of not only diabetes but also hypertension, Dyslipidemia, central body obesity and hyperinsulinaemia, all of which are part of the insulin resistance syndrome or metabolic syndrome.

A Few Things about Physical Activity

➢ It's important to be active. Physical activity has many benefits. It can help you control your blood glucose and your weight. Physical activity can help prevent heart and blood flow problems. Many people say they feel better when they get regular exercise.

➢ Start with a little. If you haven't been doing any physical activity, talk to your health care team before you begin. Walking, working in the yard, and dancing are good ways to start.

As you become stronger, you can add a few extra minutes to your physical activity. If you feel pain, slow down or stop and wait until it goes away. If the pain comes back, talk with your health care team right away.

➤ Do some physical activity every day. It's better to walk 10 or 20 minutes each day than one hour once a week.

➤ Choose an activity you enjoy. Do an activity you really like. The more fun it is, the more likely you will do it each day. It's also good to exercise with a family member or friend.

➤ Brisk walk is an activity almost everyone can do.

➤ If you're already active now, but want to become more active, talk to your health care team about a safe exercise plan.

A Few Things about Diabetes Medicine

Oral hypoglycemic agents should be used in Type 2 Diabetes in the event of failure of diet and exercise. In Unani system of Medicine certain drugs like Qurs Dolabi, Safoof Tabasheer, Qurs Ziabetus, Qurs Nashkoor, Qurs Ziabetus Khas, and Safoof Ziabetus are used, while in modern sytem of medicine various types of oral hypoglycemic agents are used like Tolbutamide, Glibenclamide, Glipizide, Metformin, and Phenformin etc. are used commonly.

If you take diabetes pills or insulin injections to control your diabetes, ask your health care provider to explain how these work. It's important to know how and when to take diabetes medicine. If you take other medicines that are sold with or without a prescription, ask your doctor how these can affect your diabetes control. When you take insulin injections or diabetes pills, your blood glucose levels can get too low.

If you inject insulin, you should be aware of:

➤ How to take injections yourself.

➤ When you need to change your insulin dose.

Be sure you know how and when to take your diabetes medicine.

Feelings about Having Diabetes

Living with diabetes isn't easy. It's normal to feel troubled about it. Tell your health care provider how you feel. Point out any problems you have with your diabetes care plan. Your diabetes educator or other health care provider may be able to help you think of ways to deal with these problems.

Family support is very helpful in managing diabetes. Talk about the stresses you feel at home, school, and work. How do you cope with these pressures? If your feelings are getting in the way of taking care of yourself, you need to ask for help.

Support Groups

It helps to talk with other people who have problems like your own. They can also talk about how they take care of their health, how they prepare food, and how they get physical activity. One-on-one and family counseling sessions may also help. Be sure to see a counselor who knows about diabetes and its care.

MANAGEMENT OF DIABETES COMPLICATIONS

EYE PROBLEMS

Diabetic eye disease (also called diabetic retinopathy) is a serious problem that can lead to loss of sight. There's a lot you can do to take charge and prevent such problems. Research shows that keeping your blood glucose level closer to normal can prevent or delay the onset of diabetic eye disease. Keeping your blood pressure under control is also important. Finding and treating eye problems early can help save sight.

> ➤ Signs of Diabetic Eye Disease

Since diabetic eye disease may be developing even when your sight is good, regular dilated eye exams are important for finding problems early. Some people may notice signs of vision changes. If you're having trouble reading, if your vision is blurred, or if you're seeing rings around lights, dark spots, or flashing lights, you may have eye problems. Be sure to tell your health care provider or eye doctor about any eye problems you may have.

> ➤ Protecting Your Sight

Keep Your Blood Glucose Under Control: High blood glucose can damage your eyes as time goes by. Keep your blood glucose levels in the target range.

Keep Your Blood Pressure Under Control: High blood pressure can damage your eyes. Have your health care provider check your blood pressure at least 4 times a year. If your blood pressure is higher than 130/80, ask your health care provider how to keep your blood pressure at a healthy level. You may need medicine to keep your blood pressure at a healthy level.

➢ Get Regular Eye Exams

Even if you're seeing fine, you need regular, complete dilated eye exams to protect your sight. Before the exam, a doctor or nurse will put drops in your eyes to dilate the pupils. You should have your eyes dilated and examined at least once a year. Even if you've lost your sight from diabetic eye disease, you still need to have regular eye care. If you haven't already had a complete eye exam, you should have one now if any of these conditions apply to you:

■ You've had type 1 diabetes for 5 or more years.

■ You have type 2 diabetes.

■ You are going through puberty and you have diabetes.

■ You are pregnant and you have diabetes.

■ You are planning to become pregnant and you have diabetes.

➢ Treating Diabetic Eye Disease

Treating eye problems early can help save sight. Laser surgery may help people who have advanced diabetic eye disease. An operation called a vitrectomy may help those who have lost their sight from bleeding in the back of the eye.

If your sight is poor, an eye doctor who is an expert in low vision may be able to give you glasses or other devices that can help you use your limited vision more fully.

KIDNEY PROBLEMS

Diabetes can cause diabetic kidney disease (also called diabetic nephropathy), which can lead to kidney failure. There's a lot you can do to take charge and prevent kidney problems. A recent study shows that controlling your blood glucose can prevent or delay the onset of kidney disease. Keeping your blood pressure under control is also important.

The kidneys keep the right amount of water in the body and help filter out harmful wastes. These wastes, called urea, then pass from the body in the urine. Diabetes can cause kidney disease by damaging the parts of the kidneys that filter out wastes. When the kidneys fail, a person has to have his or her blood filtered through a machine (a treatment called dialysis) several times a week or has to get a kidney transplant.

> ➤ Testing Your Kidneys

You can learn how well your kidneys are working by testing for microalbumin (a protein) in the urine. Microalbumin in the urine is an early sign of diabetic kidney disease. You should have your urine checked for microalbumin every year.

You can also do a yearly blood test to measure your kidney function. If the tests show microalbumin in the urine or if your kidney function isn't normal, you'll need to be checked more often.

> ➤ Protecting Your Kidneys

Keep Your Blood Glucose Under Control: High blood glucose can damage your kidneys as time goes by. Controlling your blood glucose levels and your blood pressure may help to prevent or delay kidney failure.

Keep Your Blood Pressure In Balance: High blood pressure (or hypertension) can damage your kidneys. You may want to check your blood pressure at home to be sure it stays lower than 130/80. Have your health care provider check your blood pressure at least 4 times a year. Your doctor may have you take a blood pressure pill, to help protect your kidneys.

To Lower Your Blood Pressure:

1.   Practice these steps:

■   Maintain a healthy weight.

■   Be active every day.

■   Eat fewer foods high in salt and sodium.

■   Eat more fruits and vegetables, whole grain breads and cereals, and low fat dairy products.

2.   Take your medicine the way your doctor tells you.

3.   Have your blood pressure checked often.

Call your health care provider right away if you have any of these signs of kidney infections:

■ Back pain.

■ Chills.

■ Fever.

■ Ketones in the urine.

Tell your health care provider if you have any signs of kidney or bladder infection. Your health care provider will test your urine. If you have a bladder or kidney infection, you'll be given medicine to stop the infection. After you take all the medicine, have your urine checked again to be sure the infection is gone.

> ➤ Know the Effects of Some Medicines and X-Ray Dyes

If you have kidney disease, ask your health care provider about the possible effects that some medicines and X-ray dyes can have on your kidneys.

HEART AND BLOOD VESSEL PROBLEMS

Heart and blood vessel problems are the main causes of sickness and death among people with diabetes. These problems can lead to high blood pressure, heart attacks, and strokes. Heart and blood vessel problems can also cause poor circulation (blood flow) in the legs and feet.

You're more likely to have heart and blood vessel problems if

You smoke cigarettes, have high blood pressure, or have too much cholesterol or other fats in your blood. Consult your doctor about taking a daily aspirin to help prevent heart and blood vessel problems.

> ➤ Signs of Heart and Blood Vessel Problems

If you feel dizzy, have sudden loss of sight, slur your speech, or feel numb or weak in one arm or leg, you may be having serious heart and blood vessel problems. Your blood may not be getting to your brain as well as it should. Danger signs of circulation problems to the heart include chest pain or pressure, shortness of breath, swollen ankles, or irregular heartbeats. If you have any of these signs, go to an emergency room or call your health care provider right away. Signs of circulation problems to your legs are pain or cramping in your buttocks, thighs, or calves during physical activity. Even if this pain goes away with rest, report it to your health care provider.

Preventing and Controlling Heart and Blood Vessel Problems

- Eat Right and Get Physical Activity

Choose a healthy diet, low in salt. Work with a dietitian to plan healthy meals. If you're overweight, talk about how to safely lose weight. Ask about a physical activity or exercise program for you.

- Don't Use Tobacco

Smoking cigarettes causes hundreds of thousands of deaths each year. When you have diabetes and also use tobacco, the risk of heart and blood vessel problems is even greater. One of the best choices you can make for your health is to never start smoking—or if you smoke, to quit.

- Check Your Blood Pressure

Not smoking is the healthiest choice you'll make for your heart. Get your blood pressure checked at each visit. If your blood pressure is higher than 130/80, ask what steps to take to reach your goal. If your blood pressure is still high after 3 months, you may need medicine to help control it. Many medicines are available to treat high blood pressure. If you have side effects from the medicine, ask your health care provider to change it. Talk to your health care team about whether you need medicine to take charge of your blood pressure.

- Check Your Cholesterol

Get your cholesterol checked once a year. Your total cholesterol should be lower than 200 mg/dL (milligrams per deciliter). Choose heart-healthy foods for your meal plan. If your cholesterol is higher than 200 mg/dL on two or more checks, you can do several things to lower it. You can improve your blood glucose control, you can lose weight (if you're overweight), and you can cut down on foods that are high in fat and cholesterol. Ask your doctor about foods that are low in fats. Also ask about a physical activity program.

Ask your health care provider what steps to take to reach your LDL cholesterol goal. You may need a medicine to help control it. Ask if you need aspirin to prevent heart attack or stroke.

- Ask If You Need an Electrocardiogram (EKG)

If you're having heart and blood circulation problems, an EKG may help you and your health care provider know if you need to change your treatment.

NERVE DAMAGE

Diabetic nerve damage (also called diabetic neuropathy) is a problem for many people with diabetes. Over time, high blood glucose levels damage the delicate coating of nerves. This damage can cause many problems, such as pain in your feet. There's a lot you can do to take charge and prevent nerve damage. A recent study shows that controlling your blood glucose can help prevent or delay these problems. Controlling your blood glucose may also help reduce the pain from some types of nerve damage.

➤ Some Signs of Diabetic Nerve Damage

Some signs of diabetic nerve damage are pain, burning, tingling, or loss of feeling in the feet and hands. It can cause you to sweat abnormally, make it hard for you to tell when your blood

46

glucose is low, and make you feel light-headed when you stand up. Nerve damage can lead to other problems. Some people develop problems swallowing and keeping food down. Nerve damage can also cause bowel problems, make it hard to urinate, cause dribbling. Tell your health care provider if you have trouble with sexual function. Many people with nerve damage have trouble having sex. For example, men can have trouble keeping their penis erect, a problem called impotence (erectile dysfunction). If you have any of these problems, tell your health care provider.

> ➤ Protecting Your Nerves from Damage

Keep Your Blood Glucose in Control: High blood glucose can damage your nerves as time goes by. Keep your glucose levels as close to normal as you can.

Have a Physical Activity Plan: Physical activity or exercise may help keep some nerves healthy, such as those in your feet. Ask your health care provider about an activity that is healthy for you.

At least once a year, your health care provider should do a complete check of your feet and nerves.

Get Tested for Nerve Damage: Nerve damage can happen slowly. You may not even be aware you're losing feeling in your feet. Ask your health care provider to check your feet at each visit. Your provider should test how well you can sense temperature, pinprick, vibration, and position in your feet. If you have signs of nerve damage, your provider may want to do more tests. Testing can help your provider know what is wrong and how to treat it.

Check Your Feet for Changes: If you've lost feeling in your feet, you'll need to take special care of them. Check your feet each day. Wear shoes that fit well.

FOOT PROBLEMS

Nerve damage, circulation problems, and infections can cause serious foot problems for people with diabetes. There's a lot you can do to prevent problems with your feet. Controlling your blood glucose and not smoking or using tobacco can help protect your feet. You can also take some simple safeguards each day to care for and protect your feet. Over half of diabetes-related amputations can be prevented with regular exams and patient education.

It's helpful to understand why foot problems happen. Nerve damage can cause you to lose feeling in your feet. Sometimes nerve damage can deform or misshape your feet, causing pressure points that can turn into blisters, sores, or ulcers. Poor circulation can make these injuries slow to heal.

➤ Signs of Foot Problems

Your feet may tingle, burn, or hurt. You may not be able to feel touch, heat, or cold very well. The shape of your feet can change over time. There may even be changes in the color and temperature of your feet. Some people lose hair on their toes, feet, and lower legs. The skin on your feet may be dry and cracked. Toenails may turn thick and yellow. Fungus infections can grow between your toes. Blisters, sores, ulcers, infected corns, and ingrown toenails need to be seen by your health care provider or foot doctor (podiatrist) right away.

➤ Protecting Your Feet

• Get Your Health Care Provider to Check Your Feet at Least 4 Times a Year

Have your sense of feeling and your pulses checked at least once a year. If you have nerve damage, deformed or misshaped feet, or a circulation problem, your feet need special care. Ask

48

your health care provider to show you how to care for your feet. Also ask if special shoes would help you.

- Check Your Feet Each Day

You may have serious foot problems yet feel no pain. Look at your feet every day to see if you have scratches, cracks, cuts, or blisters. Always check between your toes and on the bottoms of your feet. If you can't bend over to see the bottoms of your feet, use a mirror that won't break. If you can't see well, ask a family member or friend to help you. Call your health care provider at once if you have a sore on your foot. Sores can get worse quickly.

- Wash Your Feet Daily

Wash your feet every day. Dry them with care, especially between the toes. Don't soak your feet—it can dry out your skin, and dry skin can lead to infections. Rub lotion or cream on the tops and bottoms of your feet—but not between your toes. Moisture between the toes will let germs grow that could cause an infection.

- Trim Your Toenails Carefully

Trim your toenails after you've washed and dried your feet—the nails will be softer and safer to cut. Trim the nails to follow the natural curve of your toes. Don't cut into the corners. Use an emery board to smooth the edges. If you can't see well, or if your nails are thick or yellowed, get them trimmed by a family member. If you see redness around the nails, see your health care provider at once.

- Treat Corns and Calluses Gently

Don't cut corns and calluses. Ask your health care provider how to gently use a pumice stone to rub them. Don't use razor blades, corn plasters, or liquid corn or callus removers—they can damage your skin.

- Protect Your Feet from Heat and Cold

Hot water or hot surfaces are a danger to your feet. Before bathing, test the water with a bath thermometer (90° to 95°F is safe) or with your elbow. Wear shoes and socks when you walk on hot surfaces, such as beaches or the pavement around swimming pools. In summer, be sure to use sunscreen on the tops of your feet. You also need to protect your feet from the cold. In winter, wear socks and footwear such as fleece-lined boots to protect your feet. If your feet are cold at night, wear socks. Don't use hot water bottles, heating pads, or electric blankets—they can burn your feet. Don't use strong antiseptic solutions or adhesive tape on your feet.

- Always Wear Shoes and Socks

Wear shoes and socks at all times. Don't walk barefoot—not even indoors. Wear shoes that fit well and protect your feet. Don't wear shoes that have plastic uppers, and don't wear sandals with thongs between the toes. Ask your health care provider what types of shoes are good choices for you. New shoes should be comfortable at the time you buy them—don't expect them to stretch out. Slowly break in new shoes by wearing them only 1 or 2 hours a day. Always wear socks or stockings with your shoes. Choose socks made of cotton or wool—they help keep your feet dry. Before you put on your shoes each time, look and feel inside them. Check for any loose objects, nail points, torn linings, and rough areas—these can cause injuries. If your shoes aren't smooth inside, wear other shoes.

- Be Physically Active

Physical activity can help increase the circulation in your feet. There are many ways you can exercise your feet, even during times you're not able to walk. Ask your health care provider about things you can do to exercise your feet and legs.

DENTAL DISEASE

Because of high blood glucose, people with diabetes are more likely to have problems with their teeth and gums. There's a lot you can do to take charge and prevent these problems. Caring for your teeth and gums every day can help keep them healthy. Keeping your blood glucose under control is also important. Regular, complete dental care helps prevent dental disease.

➢ Signs of Dental Disease

Sore, swollen, and red gums that bleed when you brush your teeth are signs of a dental problem called gingivitis. Another problem, called periodontitis, happens when your gums shrink or pull away from your teeth. Like all infections, dental infections can make your blood glucose go up.

➢ Preventing Dental Problems

- Keep Your Blood Glucose Under Control

High blood glucose can cause problems with your teeth and gums. Keep your glucose levels as close to normal as you can.

- Brush Your Teeth Often

Brush your teeth at least twice a day to prevent gum disease and tooth loss. Be sure to brush before you go to sleep. Use a soft toothbrush and toothpaste with fluoride. To help keep bacteria from growing on your toothbrush, rinse it after each brushing and store it upright with the bristles at the top. Get a new toothbrush at least every 3 months.

- Floss Your Teeth Daily

Besides brushing, you need to floss between your teeth each day to help remove plaque, a film that forms on teeth and can cause tooth problems. Flossing also helps keep your gums healthy. Your dentist or dental hygienist will help you choose a good method to remove plaque, such as dental floss, bridge cleaners, or water spray. If you're not sure of the right way to brush or floss, ask your dentist for help.

- Get Regular Dental Care

Get your teeth cleaned and checked at your dentist's at least once every 6 months. See your dentist right away if you have trouble chewing or any signs of dental disease, including bad breath, a bad taste in your mouth, bleeding or sore gums, red or swollen gums, or sore or loose teeth. Plan dental visits so they don't change the times you take your insulin and meals. Don't skip a meal or diabetes medicine before your visit. Right after breakfast may be a good time for your visit.

PREGNANCY AND DIABETES

Women with diabetes can have healthy babies, but it takes planning ahead and effort. Pregnancy can make both high and low blood glucose levels happen more often. It can make diabetic eye disease and diabetic kidney disease worse. High glucose levels during pregnancy are dangerous for the baby, too.

- ➢ Protecting Your Baby and Yourself

Keeping your glucose levels near normal before and during pregnancy can help protect you and your baby. That's why it's so important to plan your pregnancies ahead of time. Your blood glucose and A1C records will help you and your health care provider know when your glucose range is safe for pregnancy. If you want to have a baby, discuss it with your health care provide. Keep your blood glucose in the normal or near-normal range before you become pregnant. Your glucose records and your A1C test results will show when you have maintained a safe range for a period of time. You may need to change your meal plan and your usual physical activity, and you may need to take more frequent insulin shots. Testing your glucose several times a day will help you see how well you are balancing things. Get a complete check of your eyes and kidneys before you try to become pregnant. Don't smoke, drink alcohol, or use drugs—doing these things can harm you and your baby. All women who could become pregnant should take folic acid (400 micrograms) every day. An easy way to be sure you're getting enough folic acid is to take a vitamin with folic acid in it. Think about breast feeding your baby. Breast feeding has many benefits for you and your baby.

➢ Having Diabetes During Pregnancy

Some women have diabetes only when they're pregnant. This condition, which is called gestational diabetes, can be controlled just like other kinds of diabetes. Glucose control is the key. You are more likely to develop type 2 diabetes. Check again for diabetes at least 6 weeks after your baby is born and at regular times for the rest of your life.

➢ Controlling Diabetes for Women's Health

Some women with diabetes may have special problems, such as bladder infections. If you have an infection, it needs to be treated right away. Call your doctor. Some women get yeast infections in their vagina, especially when their blood glucose is high. A sign of a yeast infection may be itching in the vagina. If you notice vaginal itching, tell your health care provider, who can tell you about medicines you can take and about how to prevent yeast infections. Some women with diabetes may have trouble with sexual function. Discomfort caused by vaginal itching or dryness can be treated. Regular Pap smears and mammograms help detect cervical and breast cancer early. All women—whether or not they have diabetes—need to have these tests regularly.

POINTS TO REMEMBER FOR A DIABETIC

➢ Diabetes is when your blood glucose, also called blood sugar, is too high. Blood glucose is the main type of sugar found in your blood and your main source of energy.

➢ Prediabetes is when the amount of glucose in your blood is above normal yet not high enough to be called diabetes.

➢ In type 1 diabetes, your body no longer makes insulin or enough insulin.

➢ Type 2 diabetes develops when, over time, the pancreas doesn't make enough insulin when blood sugar levels increase, such as after meals.

➢ People who are overweight and inactive are more likely to develop type 2 diabetes.

➢ Gestational diabetes can develop when a woman is pregnant. Pregnant women make hormones that can lead to insulin resistance.

➢ Gestational diabetes most often goes away after the baby is born.

➢ Do four things each day to help your blood glucose levels stay in your target range:

• Follow your healthy eating plan.

• Be physically active.

• Take your medicines as prescribed.

• Monitor your diabetes.

➢ People with diabetes should aim for 30 to 60 minutes of activity most days of the week. Children and adolescents with type 2 diabetes who are 10 to 17 years old should aim for 60 minutes of activity every day.

➢ Check your blood glucose levels before, during, and after physical activity.

➢ Your doctor may prescribe you diabetes medicines that work best for you and your lifestyle.

➢ If you have type 1 diabetes, you need insulin shots if your body has stopped making insulin or if it doesn't make enough. Some people with type 2 diabetes or gestational diabetes also need to take insulin shots.

➢ Ask your health care provider when you should take your diabetes medicines.

➢ Checking and recording your blood glucose levels can help you monitor and better manage your diabetes. Ask your doctor how often you should check your blood glucose levels.

➢ You may need to check your blood or urine for ketones if you're sick or if your blood glucose levels are above 240

➢ If your blood glucose levels stay above 180 for more than 1 to 2 hours, they may be too high. High blood glucose, also called hyperglycemia, means you don't have enough insulin in your body.

➢ If your blood glucose levels drop below 70, you have low blood glucose, also called hypoglycemia.

➢ If you take diabetes medicines that can cause low blood glucose, always carry food for emergencies.

➢ If you take insulin, keep a prescription glucagon kit at home and at other places where you often go. If you have severe hypoglycemia, you'll need someone to help bring your blood glucose levels back to normal by giving you a glucagon shot.

➤ Tell your teachers, friends, or close coworkers that you have diabetes and teach them about the signs of low blood glucose. You may need their help if your blood glucose levels drop too low.

➤ Get all your vaccines and immunizations, or shots, before you travel. Find out what shot you need for where you're going, and make sure you get the right shots on time.

➤ When traveling, carry your diabetes medicines and your blood testing supplies with you on the plane. Never put these items in your checked baggage.

➤ Keeping your blood glucose levels near normal before and during pregnancy helps protect both you and your baby.

GLOSSARY

A1C — A test that sums up how much glucose has been sticking to part of the hemoglobin during the past 3–4 months. Hemoglobin is a substance in the red blood cells that supplies oxygen to the cells of the body. The AIC goal for patients in general is an AIC goal of less than 7%. The AIC goal for the individual patient is an AIC as close to 6% as possible without a considerable amount of low blood glucose.

Autoimmune process — A process where the body's immune system attacks and destroys body tissue that it mistakes for foreign matter.

Beta cells — Cells that make insulin. Beta cells are found in areas of the pancreas called the Islets of Langerhans.

Bladder — A hollow organ that urine drains into from the kidneys. From the bladder, urine leaves the body.

Blood glucose — The main sugar that the body makes from the food we eat. Glucose is carried through the bloodstream to provide energy to all of the body's living cells. The cells cannot use glucose without the help of insulin.

Calluses — Thick, hardened areas of the skin, generally on the foot, caused by friction or pressure. Calluses can lead to other problems, including serious infection and even gangrene.

Carbohydrate — One of three main groups of foods in the diet that provide calories and energy. (Protein and fat are the others.) Carbohydrates are mainly sugars (simple carbohydrates) and starches (complex carbohydrates, found in bread, pasta, beans) that the body breaks down into glucose.

Cholesterol — A substance similar to fat that is found in the blood, muscles, liver, brain, and other body tissues. The body produces and needs some cholesterol. However, too much cholesterol can make fats stick to the walls of the arteries and cause a disease that decreases or stops circulation.

Chronic kidney disease (CKD) — retains fluids and harmul wastes build up because the kidneys no longer work properly.

Corns — A thickening of the skin of the feet or hands, usually caused by pressure against the skin.

Dehydration — the loss of too much body fluid through frequent urinating, sweating, diarrhea, or vomiting.

Diabetes — The short name for the disease called diabetes mellitus. Diabetes results when the body cannot use blood glucose as energy because of having too little insulin or being unable to use insulin. See also type 1 diabetes, type 2 diabetes, and gestational diabetes.

Diabetes pills — Pills or capsules that are taken by mouth to help lower the blood glucose level. These pills may work for people whose bodies are still making insulin.

Diabetic eye disease — A disease of the small blood vessels of the retina of the eye in people with diabetes. In this disease, the vessels swell and leak liquid into the retina, blurring the vision and sometimes leading to blindness.

Diabetic ketoacidosis — High blood glucose with the presence of ketones in the urine and bloodstream, often caused by taking too little insulin or during illness.

Diabetic kidney disease — Damage to the cells or blood vessels of the kidney.

Diabetic nerve damage — Damage to the nerves of a person with diabetes. Nerve damage may affect the feet and hands, as well as major organs.

Dialysis — A method for removing waste from the blood when the kidneys can no longer do the job.

Dilated eye exam — Eye drops are placed in the eyes to widen the pupils to see the retina better. The eye doctor will look for changes in the retinain the back of the eyes.

EKG — A test that measures the heart's action. Also called an electrocardiogram.

Gestational diabetes — A type of diabetes that can occur in pregnant women who have not been known to have diabetes before.

GFR (Glumerular filration rate) - A measure of the kidney's ability to filter and remove waste products. It is the best tst to measure kidney function and stage of kidney disease.

Gingivitis — A swelling and soreness of the gums that, without treatment, can cause serious gum problems and disease.

Glucagon — A hormone that raises the blood glucose level.

Glucose — A sugar in our blood and a source of energy for our bodies.

Heart attack — Damage to the heart muscle caused when the blood vessels supplying the muscle are blocked, such as when the blood vessels are clogged with fats (a condition sometimes called hardening of the arteries).

HDL (or high-density lipoprotein) — A combined protein and fatlike substance. Low in cholesterol, it usually passes freely through the arteries. Sometimes called "good cholesterol."

High blood glucose — A condition that occurs in people with diabetes when their blood glucose levels are too high. Symptoms include having to urinate often, being very thirsty, and losing weight.

High blood pressure — A condition where the blood circulates through the arteries with too much force. High blood pressure tires the heart, harms the arteries, and increases the risk of heart attack, stroke, and kidney problems.

Hormone — A chemical that special cells in the body release to help other cells work. For example, insulin is a hormone made in the pancreas to help the body use glucose as energy.

Immunization — Sometimes called vaccination; a shot or injection that protects a person from getting an illness by making the person "immune" to it.

Insulin — A hormone that helps the body use blood glucose for energy. The beta cells of the pancreas make insulin. When people with diabetes can't make enough insulin, they may have to inject it from another source.

Ketones — Chemical substances that the body makes when it doesn't have enough insulin in the blood. When ketones build up in the body for a long time, serious illness or coma can result.

Kidneys — Twin organs found in the lower part of the back. The kidneys purify the blood of all waste and harmful material. They also control the level of some helpful chemical substances in the blood.

Laser surgery — Surgery that uses a strong ray of special light, called a laser, to treat damaged parts of the body. Laser surgery can help treat some diabetic eye diseases.

Low blood glucose — A condition that occurs in people with diabetes when their blood glucose levels are too low. Symptoms include feeling anxious or confused, feeling numb in the arms and hands, and shaking or feeling dizzy.

LDL (or low-density lipoprotein) — A combined protein and fatlike substance. Rich in cholesterol, it tends to stick to the walls in the arteries. Sometimes called "bad cholesterol".

Meal plan — A guide to help people get the proper amount of calories, carbohydrates, proteins, and fats in their diet. See also food exchanges.

Microalbumin — A protein found in blood plasma and urine. The presence of microalbumin in the urine can be a sign of kidney disease.

Nephropathy — See diabetic kidney disease.

Neuropathy — See diabetic nerve damage.

Non–insulin-dependent diabetes — See type 2 diabetes.

Pancreas — An organ in the body that makes insulin so that the body can use glucose for energy. The pancreas also makes enzymes that help the body digest food.

Periodontitis — A gum disease in which the gums shrink away from the teeth. Without treatment, it can lead to tooth loss.

Plaque — A film of mucus that traps bacteria on the surface of the teeth. Plaque can be removed with daily brushing and flossing of teeth.

Risk factors — Traits that make it more likely that a person will get an illness. For example, a risk factor for getting type 2 diabetes is having a family history of diabetes.

Self-monitoring blood glucose — A way for people with diabetes to find out how much glucose is in their blood. A drop of blood from the fingertip is placed on a special coated strip of paper that "reads" (often through an electronic meter) the amount of glucose in the blood.

Stroke — Damage to a part of the brain that happens when the blood vessels supplying that part are blocked, such as when the blood vessels are clogged with fats (a condition sometimes called hardening of the arteries).

Type 1 diabetes — A condition in which the pancreas makes so little insulin that the body can't use blood glucose as energy. People with type 1 diabetes need to take insulin every day.

Type 2 diabetes — A condition in which the body either makes too little insulin or can't use the insulin it makes to use blood glucose as energy. All people with diabetes need to eat healthy foods stay at a healthy weight and be active everyday. People with type 2 often need to diabetes have to take diabetes pills or insulin. type 2 diabetes is the most common form of diabetes.

Ulcer — A break or deep sore in the skin. Germs can enter an ulcer and may be hard to heal.

Urea — One of the chief waste product of the body. When the body breaks down food, it uses what it needs and throws the rest away as waste. The kidneys flush the waste from the body in the form of urea, which is in the urine.

Vaccination — A shot given to protect against a disease.

Vagina — A canal in females from the external genitalia (vulva) to the cervix of the uterus.

Vitrectomy — An operation to remove the blood that sometimes collects at the back of the eyes when a person has eye disease.

Yeast infection — A vaginal infection that is usually caused by a fungus. Women who have this infection may feel itching, burning when urinating, and pain, and some women have a vaginal discharge. Yeast infections occur more frequently in women with diabetes.

www.ingramcontent.com/pod-product-compliance
Lightning Source LLC
Chambersburg PA
CBHW040837180526
45159CB00001B/218

* 9 7 8 1 5 1 6 9 7 8 9 8 4 *